Lymphedema

Finding the Holistic Approach

Phillip J. Pollot, L.M.T. and C.D.T.

Do not drink ē meals
Plain yogurt (with fruits)
Drink tepid water upon waking

To my wife Eileen,
my inspiration
in my search;
and to all of my
lymphedema clients,
who teach and encourage me
to discover new pathways
to lymphatic health.

2 oz. grape juice
4 oz. water
1/2 Hr. before meals
+ @ bed time
2-3 x wk.
for 4-6 wks. Then stop
for 2-3 wks. Then start
again.

Cover illustration by Miriam M. Zaffrann Thanks to Sandra Duggan, R.N., for information on colonic irrigation.

MLD® is a trademark of the North American Vodder Association of Lymphatic Therapists.

Throughout this book, reference is made to various Edgar Cayce Readings; the numbers that appear after each reference represent the actual Edgar Cayce reading numbers.

First published by Dog Ear Publishing
4010 W. 86th Street, Ste H
Indianapolis, IN 46268
www.dogearpublishing.net

dog ear
PUBLISHING

ISBN: 978-160844-557-8

Therapy Comments

The single most important aspect of dealing with lymphedema has been knowing that I have control over it – I couldn't have lived with breast cancer, but I can live, and live well, with lymphedema by eating correctly, exercising in moderation, and by getting regular massage, manual lymph drainage and other therapies. I feel better now than I have in years!

E.S.

I'd reached a plateau with my leg lymphedema and I wanted more. Phillip Pollot's program is getting results. My leg is tauter, smaller, and better functioning. I am dancing again. Food combining makes a dramatic difference in reducing lymphedema and helping me move with joy. I feel optimistic and in charge of my lymphedema.

M.L.B.

Upon meeting Phil, I felt like he was the first person I met who had a 360-degree grasp of lymphedema and its impact on a person's life. No one, not my oncologist, surgeon, radiation oncologist or even the physical therapists – treated it as anything more than an annoying side effect of the bigger disease. In addition to providing hour-long intensive Manual Lymph Drainage, Phil counseled me in nutrition, and its impact on both lymphedema and cancer. After seven sessions with Phil, my arm has never felt better. For once I could blend into a crowd of strangers without hearing, "What did you do to your arm?" This is a huge step toward shedding the "cancer victim" image. I never dreamed that my condition could be managed down to a level of virtual normalcy. I firmly believe that physical manipulation is not enough to combat this stubborn condition. Coupling Manual Lymph Drainage with a sound diet has boosted me to a new level of wellness.

J.T.

Physical therapy had brought the swelling down in my arm, but I had persistent swelling in my hand and minimal success with it. During a consult with Phil we discussed dietary considerations that may be influencing my lymphedema. We concentrated on increasing my vegetables, especially leafy greens, and decreasing my starch and protein. We also eliminated refined flour and sugar, diet sodas and decreased my coffee intake. I saw an immediate reduction in the swelling in my hand and was able to maintain that when I stayed on the diet. We then used the Light Beam Generator on the remaining edema. After 3 or 4 sessions I again saw an improvement in the edema in my hand. My hand is now very close to my normal size, and I am able to maintain it by self-management.

L.O.

The most important aspects of my treatments were the Manual Lymph Drainage treatments and the dietary changes. Through the use of compression and my husband's help with massage, my arm edema is controlled and I am able to go about freely.

I.M.

In the spring of 2000, I suffered my first infection in my right leg. Once the infection was resolved, I was left with a severely swollen and hard right leg. The doctors offered no source of resolution other than compression stockings. I was told that this was a condition I would have to live with, and that was that. I began my search for alternative resolutions to the problem. With the help of local contacts, I found Phil Pollot. Phil has helped me with both Manual Lymph Drainage and diet. With his help and guidance, I have lost 30 pounds. The effect of reducing the fat in both my diet and body has been to bring my leg problems under control. I not only personally feel better, but my leg is better.

D.B.

Table of Contents

All knowledge is to be used in the manner that will give help and assistance to others.

-Edgar Cayce

Introduction

My interest in lymphedema and in the possibility of treating it with alternative therapies began after my wife underwent treatment for breast cancer. Her treatment involved a lumpectomy with axillary dissection and radiation therapy. Shortly after her treatment she developed lymphedema of the arm. We were aware of the limited success that the medical community had up to that point in alleviating the symptoms of lymphedema (if those symptoms were addressed at all), and began to research other options.

Approximately 240,000 new cases of breast cancer were diagnosed in the United States in 2007 alone (American Cancer Society). Increasing numbers of women go on to live long, productive lives after treatment. Unfortunately, the side effects of breast cancer treatment can be long-lasting and in themselves quality of life issues, and as such need to be addressed by the healing community.

One of the more common side effects of breast cancer treatment is lymphedema of the arm, which is the chronic accumulation of fluid in the tissues. The risk for developing lymphedema depends upon the extent of surgery and radiation treatment, and on whether or not there was axillary lymph node removal.

Lymphedema can also develop in a leg after pelvic surgery or radiation therapy, and can also arise from congenital conditions. Lymphedema can be treated successfully in a number of ways, including Manual Lymph Drainage, compression garments, "friendly food" considerations, light therapy, and remedial exercise.

At the time of my wife's diagnosis with lymphedema, I was

completing my training in massage therapy. It was only natural that I look to alternative medicine for viable treatment options. I explored the different treatment techniques being used throughout the world, and became interested in the Vodder Manual Lymph Drainage System, a type of massage successfully used to treat compromised lymphatic systems for decades. I became certified as a Combined Decongestive Therapist from the Vodder School, and my wife became my first patient.

In addition to Manual Lymph Drainage® (MLD), her treatment included the use of compression garments, an exercise program, and Light Beam Generator® therapy (LBG). She has also found significant improvement (to the point where she does not need to wear a compression sleeve) by changing her diet to "friendly" foods, adapted from Edgar Cayce's holistic health readings.

I have since gone on to treat a variety of clients suffering from lymphedema, using the same techniques with which my wife had such success. My clients have experienced varying degrees of improvement, confirming my belief that lymphedema, when approached on a holistic level, can be successfully treated.

This book contains a basic overview of the program I teach my clients. I believe it can offer a degree of relief from even the most stubborn cases of lymphedema. While each component of the program, in itself, is beneficial in treating lymphedema, the highest degree of success can be found through incorporating all aspects of the program.

I encourage you to embrace the information in this book to make a difference in your lymphedema and the quality of your life.

Phillip J. Pollot, LMT CDT

No one succeeds without effort...Those who succeed owe their success to their perseverance.

-Famana Maharshi

The Lymphatic System

The **lymphatic system** is made up of lymph (a clear fluid), lymph vessels and lymph nodes. Its function is to collect *excess fluid, proteins, fats, inorganics and organics* from the tissues, filter it, and return it to the bloodstream. It plays an important role in protecting us against disease and illness.

Lymph consists of fluid collected from the space between tissue cells. It travels from the tissue spaces, through lymphatic vessels, to lymph nodes located throughout the body, where it is filtered and cleaned. Once it leaves the lymph nodes, it continues through the larger lymphatic vessels, the thoracic duct and right and left lymphatic vessels, to the subclavian veins, where it is returned to the bloodstream. The lymphatic vessels that initially collect the fluid from tissue cells are called capillaries, and they are open-ended, moving the fluid from the tissues into the capillary and then on to the next section of the vessels. Small valves prevent the lymph fluid from flowing back. The lymph fluid moves as our skeletal muscles contract, through arterial pulsation, diaphragmatic breathing and peristaltic action.

The lymphatic system absorbs the excess fluid that is not reabsorbed by the veins. Normally, the veins reabsorb approximately 90% of the fluid in the tissues, and the lymph vessels transport the remaining 10%. This fluid is referred to as the lymph obligatory load (LOL). In times of stress or trauma, the lymphatic system transports a much larger quantity of fluid. One example of this is when a person engages in heavy exercise. Another is in cases of edema. **Edema** results from an unbalanced ratio of fluid entering tissue and exiting the lymphatic system, causing an abnormal amount of fluid to collect in the tissues. It is often symptomatic of an underlying disorder.

Lymphedema occurs when the ability of the lymphatic system to transport fluid has been compromised, resulting in an accumulation of protein-rich fluid in the tissue spaces. This excess fluid causes swelling, which decreases the oxygenation of the tissues and interferes with normal cell function. As the lymph stagnates in the tissues, it provides an excellent medium for bacterial growth, increasing the risk of infection. If the protein-rich fluid remains in the tissues, the excess proteins will begin to align, causing a thickening of tissue (fibrosis).

There are two main causes of lymphedema: primary (congenital) and secondary:

Primary/congenital lymphedema usually affects one limb, and most commonly occurs in females. In primary/congenital lymphedema, the lymph vessels are unable to efficiently transport the lymph fluid. There may be an inadequate number of lymph vessels, or vessels that are too large and have back flow prevention valves that function improperly. This condition can appear at birth, at puberty, or later in life.

Secondary lymphedema can result from many conditions, including surgery, radiation therapy, accidental trauma, chronic venous insufficiency, re-occurring infections in a limb, parasites (common in tropical countries), post-operative infections, plastic surgery and liposuction. Breast cancer treatment, especially that which involves the removal of lymph nodes, is the number-one cause. Men treated for prostate cancer, or women treated for gynecologic cancer with inguinal node dissection or radiation may also suffer from lymphedema, primarily in the lower limbs.

Vodder Manual Lymph Drainage

In 1932, Dr. Emil Vodder and his wife, Dr. Estrid Vodder, were working as massage therapists in Cannes on the French Riviera. Most of their clients were English and were there to recover from chronic colds, thought to be caused by the damp climate in Britain. During the course of working with clients in their Physical Therapy Institute, the Vodders were struck by the fact that the majority of them had swollen lymph nodes in their necks. One client in particular caused Emil Vodder to turn this observation into a hypothesis. The client had come to them with a nose and throat infection, migraine, and blemished, oily skin. His lymph nodes were hard and swollen. While working on the client, Dr. Vodder suddenly came to understand the lymphatic system as a natural separate drainage apparatus for the entire head region and it became obvious to him that obstructed, and therefore malfunctioning, lymph nodes could only lead to a host of symptoms and ailments. He immediately began to wonder if he could unblock this drainage system with specific massage treatments.

At that time the lymphatic system was taboo not only for massage therapists but for physicians as well. It was poorly understood and was regarded as a medical Pandora's box. Massaging the lymph nodes was especially discouraged as those in the medical community believed that such treatment would only spread bacteria and viruses. Mistaken beliefs such as these about the lymphatic system lead to the prevailing practice of ignoring it completely. Vodder dared to break this taboo and began treating swollen lymph nodes intuitively and successfully. The colds and other symptoms vanished. Encouraged by their successes, Drs. Emil and Estrid Vodder went on to develop a simple systematic list of massage movements based on their extensive practical experience, which became the Manual Lymph Drainage method as it is taught and applied today.

First introduced to the public in Paris in spring of 1936, the Manual Lymph Drainage method is now used throughout the world. After coining the term and establishing their place in medical history as the originators of this unique and invaluable treatment tool, the Vodders made it their life work to teach others about their remarkable discovery. For forty years, they remained active as massage therapists, lecturers, and teachers. This work continues at the Vodder Society for Dr. Vodder's Lymph Drainage in Austria, established in 1972, where the unaltered, original method is taught by certified instructors. Vodder courses are also taught at different institutions located in various parts of the world by teachers who have undergone training and become certified in the Manual Lymph Drainage method.

MLD techniques can be beneficial not only in the treatment of lymphedema, but also in the treatment of a variety of other ailments. Thirty years of research in Europe has documented these benefits and MLD is commonly prescribed by European physicians, who recognize that the removal of excess fluid expedites the healing process, and can be used in as many as sixty different indications. MLD techniques can also benefit healthy people by stimulating the lymphatic system, causing it to carry away excess fluids and allowing the body tissues to assimilate nutrients quicker. It also expedites the removal of cellular by-products and any toxins that may be present. A few of the indications that MLD can be used for are:

Surgical

Pre- and Post- surgery edemas
Mastectomy edema
Hysterectomy edema
Dental and sinus surgery

Dermatological

Acne
Eczema
Diabetic ulcers
Burns

Musculoskeletal

Sprains and Fractures
Severe whiplash injuries

Neurological

Migraines, Tension headaches
Neuralgia
Reflex sympathetic dystrophy
Carpal tunnel syndrome

**Knowledge of what is possible is the
beginning of happiness.**
- George Santayanna

Light Beam Generator Therapy

The Light Beam Generator (LBG) is a noninvasive handheld instrument that functions to restore healthy lymph function and help eliminate wastes. While it has been used to treat a wide range of conditions, including sciatica, PMS, inflammation, skin problems, allergies, arthritis, diabetes, fibromyalgia and fibrocystic disease, the Light Beam Generator is best used for reducing or eliminating edema, including lymphedema, sometimes in as little as one session. Whatever condition it is used to treat, the Light Beam Generator's success lies in its ability to improve lymph flow, thus enhancing the delivery of oxygen and vital nutrients throughout the bloodstream. It is also able to kill fungus, bacteria, and viruses that feed on pooled wastes in the lymphatic system.

Developed by ELF International, the LBG works to reduce lymphedema by breaking up clumps of cells in the lymphatic system through the use of low-current, cold gas light photons. While similar to laser therapy, another light-based technology, it is a gentler approach and can be used safely by lay practitioners.

Cells have an electromagnetic charge that can either bind them together or keep them apart. The congestion found in the lymphatic system include damaged proteins, which are characterized by instability. The job of the lymphatic system is to remove these proteins from the body before they can cause any problems. However, when the lymphatic system is congested and not functioning properly, these proteins remain in the lymph fluid for a longer period of time than is healthy, and have a tendency to attract and bond with water. The result of these clumps of water-retaining cells is edema.

The LBG breaks up these cell masses by targeting the unhealthy protein structures and changing each cell's electromagnetic charge, causing it to separate from the water instead of bond with it. Once this bond is broken, the Vodder Manual Lymph Drainage method is used to move the water and proteins back into the circulatory system, where the body can process these wastes to restore normal body function.

To obtain long-lasting results, it is recommended that this therapy be combined with MLD, compression, "friendly food" considerations and exercise. Approaching the treatment process on a holistic level increases the likelihood that optimum results will be achieved.

Dietary Considerations

In addition to the use of Manual Lymph Drainage and Light Beam Generator therapy, the foods we ingest are an important component in creating and maintaining a healthy lymphatic system. Eating whole foods that are low in fat and protein, with an emphasis on fruits and vegetables, has been shown to reduce the effects of lymphedema. By building your meals around vegetables and fruits, you also help lighten the workload of the lymphatic system. Special consideration needs to be made for calcium intake (both amount and type), adequate vitamin D consumption, the reduction of acid-forming foods, and the amount of fluids taken in. Making these changes will greatly improve the health of your lymphatic system.

The Calcium / Protein Connection

Since the healthy flow of lymph is dependent on calcium, maintaining appropriate levels of this mineral is critical. The tendency is to do this by drinking milk and eating dairy products, but this can do more harm than good. For years, it has been assumed that since dairy itself is high in calcium, incorporating milk products into meals will lead to increased levels of calcium in the body. A number of high-profile studies have recently led many to question this theory, and to look at the role of protein, in which dairy is naturally high, in calcium retention.

The largest study to look at the relationship between dairy consumption and bone health is the ongoing Nurses Health Study, in which 78,000 women have been followed over a 12-year period. Recent calculations show no evidence that women consuming one to three servings daily of dairy have any reduction in hip fractures, the standard measure for osteoporosis (thought to be caused by insufficient calcium). The same holds true for women consuming more than three servings per day. In fact, those who drink the most milk are the ones most likely to have broken a hip. And the nurses who consume the most protein overall (more that 95 grams per day) have a 22% higher risk of arm fracture than those who eat less than 68 grams per day.

Epidemiological studies show that worldwide, dairy intake is correlated with an increase in fractures from osteoporosis. In addition to this, the incidence of bone fractures rises in areas where protein intake, specifically that from animals, is highest. Studies show that women living in Peru, Ceylon, Central America, and Africa maintain healthy bones on 200 to 475 milligrams daily (compared to our RDA of 1200 milligrams). The explanation for this may be fairly simple, in light of the emerging research on calcium intake and its use in the body.

It has become apparent that maintaining adequate levels of calcium in the body depends not so much on how much calcium is taken in, but on how much calcium is lost through urine, sweat, and feces. One of the key factors influencing calcium loss is high protein intake, causing us to question the standard American high-protein diet, which includes our consumption of dairy products.

Protein, from the Greek word *proteios*, meaning of *first importance,* is a critical part of our diet. The normal lean adult body is approximately 12-18% protein; the body uses some of these proteins in the form of enzymes to speed up biochemical reactions, others as the machinery for muscle contraction and still others as hormones. Protein is also necessary for the synthesis of new proteins.

The problem with protein, along with a number of other foods, is that it creates an acidic condition in the body, which constantly seeks to maintain a blood pH between 7.35 and 7.45. When the blood becomes too acidic, calcium is leached from the skeletal system and into the bloodstream, where it acts to restore the appropriate acid-alkaline balance. Over time, this can create a calcium shortage, resulting in a reduction in the amount of calcium available to the smooth muscles controlling lymph flow, which in turn affects the muscle's peristaltic motion. (See page 23 for more on the acid/alkalizing connection.)

According to Neal Bernard, M.D., clinical researcher and president of the Physicians Committee for Responsible Medicine, you can cut your calcium losses in half by eliminating animal protein from your diet and by avoiding food combinations that create even greater acidic conditions in the body. The lower a person's protein intake, the lower their calcium needs. And these needs can generally be met by eating plant-based foods.

Protein is made up of amino acids, some of which are essential, meaning that we need to get them from our food, and others that are non-essential, which means that the body is capable of producing them. Animal products provide complete proteins; which means that they contain all of the essential amino acids. Plant foods do not. Different plant foods provide different essential amino acids, which combine with each other throughout the day to form complete proteins. Eating a variety of plant-based foods can provide all the protein necessary for good health.

It bears mentioning, however, that individuals vary in their needs, and some people may not feel their best trying to meet all of their protein needs with plant food. Some physically active individuals may find it difficult to get all of their protein from plant sources, and may need some animal protein for optimum health.

Once the intake of animal protein is reduced, our calcium needs can easily be met by plant foods. Good sources of calcium include broccoli, collards, kale, mustard greens, okra, bok choy, winter squash, orange juice fortified with calcium, soymilk fortified with calcium, tofu coagulated with calcium, seaweeds, beans and nuts (especially almonds), figs, blackstrap molasses, sesame seeds and tahini.

Calcios - Calcium

Approximately 98% of all calcium in the average adult is located in the skeleton and teeth, combined with phosphates to form a crystal lattice - bone. Without this lattice, we would basically be blobs, much like water balloons. It is bone that gets us upright, allowing us to move about. The blood has normal concentrations of 4.6-5.5 mEq/liter of unattached free Ca, and that amount again attaching to various plasma proteins. What this means for us is that blood will clot, our nerves will be able to communicate, we will have good muscle tone, and there can be excitability of nerves and muscle tissue. In short we are free to walk or run, use our hands, think, etc.

We all know from the media that women and men need calcium to prevent osteoporosis. One in two women and one in four men will have an osteoporosis-related fracture during their lifetime. The Cayce Readings suggested adding calcium to the diet in the form of Calcios. A half-teaspoon of Calcios contains 243 mg. of predigested calcium, pancreatin, pepsin, hydrochloric acid and trace minerals including iodine. Calcios was originally manufactured by the Colloidal Health Products Corporation in Greenvale, Long Island, NY and has been mentioned in the Edgar Cayce readings beginning in 1939. This paste is now sold by the Heritage Store in Virginia Beach, Virginia, 1-800-862-2923.

The Edgar Cayce readings stated "Then the activity of the calcium or lime in the Calcios, as we find, is almost free; while much of this may be taken from vegetables, these properties will be easily assimilated, and the activity of the calcium is to produce for the blood CELLULAR forces that which adds to the EFFECTIVENESS as it were of the color and the covering of the blood CELLS themselves!" – 1548-2.

From mainstream information and from the readings we can readily see the benefits of calcium for our bodies. We know that calcium will help the lymph system function better; other readings say it "...will keep away those tendencies for colds, congestions, and overcome those conditions which have been upset by such attacks on portions of the glandular forces of the body. Also better resistance will be builded."- 1566-4. The lack of calcium can have a profound effect on circulation, especially on the smooth muscle of the lymph vessels – "a better circulation of the heart's activity will be maintained if there is sufficient quantity of calcium through the system at all times. While it makes for structural portions or build of the body itself, - that is, within, - it will be better for both." – 1505-6. Biting ones fingernail, ridges in the fingernails and teeth indicates a lack of calcium – 1958-2, 2797-1 and 5192-1. If you are suffering from broken fingernails, sluggish glands, creaking bones, fatigue and poor lymph circulation, you may need calcium. Cayce also prescribed it for a sluggish thyroid gland.

It is recommended that you take a ½ teaspoon two or three times a week. If you live in the tropics the readings suggested one or two times a week. The readings said this is the most assimilating form of calcium supplement. Cayce cautions: "Take only the quantity as may be easily spread on a whole wheat cracker, eaten at mealtime when the meal is not hurried. Don't take it all at once, for the body only assimilates so much."- 1947-8. By skipping days, the body has the chance to assimilate the calcium without causing accumulations and producing "bony structures in an abnormal manner". – 5412-1, or "accumulations around joints". – 3012-1.

As I remember from my Dr. Vodder training, there must be free calcium present for good peristaltic action of the lymph vessels. We should always remember that it is best to call on Mother Nature for our diet rather than take supplements in hopes of correcting a poor diet. We must address the foods we are eating and the combinations of foods at our meal times. To cut down on the acidity of our meals we need to be eating 60 – 80 % vegetables and fruit and complementing these with 20 – 40 % whole grains and lighter proteins. Avoid eating processed foods and eat the real thing that Mother Nature has given us. At your meals avoid protein with starch, starch with starch, and citrus with starch. Do this at least six days a week. This will allow the body to have more free calcium as it is not needed to buffer the high acid diet most people eat.

If you are seeking to increase your calcium intake, here is a list of foods rich in calcium: Spinach, steel cut oats, whole grain cereals, onions, garlic, rhubarb, raw cabbage, turnips, turnip greens, beets, celery, carrots, water cress, lettuce, citrus fruits, parsnips and oyster plant, to name a few. Calcium is available from fish bones (canned salmon) and fowl, especially the neck, head, wings and feet. It's important to remember that vitamin D works in conjunction with calcium to help the body absorb it. Vitamin D comes from exposure to sunlight; could it be that those living in the tropics with more sun exposure have less bone fractures?

You may note that I didn't mention milk or cheese as a source of calcium. Cayce did mention milk and cheese as a good source; however, the milking of cows by the American Dairy industry has dramatically changed over time. Cow's milk today has large amounts of female sex hormones and accounts for 60 to 80 percent of the estrogens consumed. Cows today are milked about 300 days a year during which most of the time the cows are pregnant. The further into the pregnancy the more hormones are present; in fact, the hormones are 33 times as much as a non-pregnant cow. In a typical herding society such as Mongolia they milk their cows only 150 days per year and not into late pregnancy. The Mongolian cow's milk has much lower levels of hormones. Their children have much lower levels of hormones than children drinking American milk. What affect on children do these hormone levels have – no one knows!

A 42 country study of prostate cancer shows that the higher the milk and cheese consumption the higher the prostate cancer rate – led by Sweden and Denmark where cheese is their national food. In Japan, fifty years ago the death rate from prostate cancer was zero; it has increased to 7 per 100,000 with the increasing consumption of dairy. Breast cancer, a hormone-dependent cancer, has been linked to dairy consumption. More studies need to be done for this controversy to have a conclusion.

American skim milk has lower levels of hormones; however, studies from T. Colin Campbell, PhD, have shown that the animal protein is so acidic that it robs the body of more calcium than it brings when ingested. In the U.S., we lead the way in cow's milk consumption and we lead the way in bone fractures; Singapore has the least bone fractures with the least milk consumption. The peristaltic action of the lymph vessels, among other body functions, is also affected by high dairy intake.

The Cayce readings described the therapeutic effects of using Calcios as a dietary supplement. Stronger tooth enamel and healthier gums, better resistance to disease, stronger blood, stronger body structure, improved circulation (in cases of low blood pressure, and poor lymph circulation), improved glandular function (thyroid), stops splitting nails, less hair loss, better pregnancy and gestation, helps in the treatment of tuberculosis, improved digestion and assimilation, better eliminations, more nerve energy, alkalizing of the body, and a better hepatic system.

Even before I knew all these benefits I was taking Calcios, it stopped my brittle nails and a splitting nail on my right hand. Calcios has helped many clients with weak nails and I hope an improvement in their lymphatic system functioning and other body functions.

Other Factors Affecting Calcium Levels

Vitamin D

Calcium absorption is dependent on adequate amounts of vitamin D, which is synthesized from sunlight and is found in limited supply in food sources. Because of the risk of sunburn, people with lymphedema are advised to limit their exposure to sunlight, especially to the affected limb. Many of the foods that contain vitamin D are also high in animal protein, and should be taken in moderation. If you are low on Vitamin D it is recommended that one teaspoon of cod liver oil be taken daily as a supplement to the meal. Non-dairy foods that are high in Vitamin D include herring, salmon, and sardines.

Caffeine, Salt, Tobacco, Alcohol, and Phosphorous

Caffeine and salt increase the amount of calcium excreted in the urine. Seventy-five percent of the salt we take in comes from processed foods, which should be avoided. Salt also encourages water retention.

Smoking, excessive alcohol consumption, and excessive fat intake interfere with the absorption of calcium. Smoking also inhibits circulation. Alcohol dehydrates the body, robbing the lymphatic system of water, its transportation vehicle.

High phosphorous intake (red meat and soft drinks) depletes bone calcium stores to maintain blood calcium-phosphorus balance.

Acid and Alkalizing Foods

Foods can be classified according to the affect they have on the body when metabolized. Some foods are distinctly acid-forming, some are alkalizing, and others are buffers, and can act as either, depending on what they are consumed with. When a diet is high in acid-forming foods, calcium is one of the minerals used as a buffering agent, necessary to restore the blood to a normal pH level. Because of the importance of calcium in maintaining a healthy lymphatic system, it is recommended that foods that are acid-forming be limited so that calcium levels in the body are not depleted. When foods that are acid-forming are consumed, it is important that alkalinizing foods be eaten in the meal to balance out the effect on the blood.

Alkalinizing foods consist of most fruits and starchless vegetables. These are the foods we need to emphasize in our meals. Fruits and starchless vegetables (these are typically vegetables that grow above the ground, including broccoli, kale, chard, etc.) should make up 60 to 80% of our nutritional intake; starch vegetables (such as sweet potatoes, parsnips, and winter squash) should be consumed 2-3 times a week.

Acid-forming foods are basically all other foods, such as whole grains, proteins, and fats. These foods should complement our alkalizing foods, comprising 20-40% of our meals. An excessively acidic state can also slow down lymph flow and lead to lymphatic congestion, causing inflammation within the lymph system and clogging the vessels and nodes.

Fluids

It is especially important to keep the body well-hydrated when dealing with lymphedema. Water is a component of lymph, and is the transport medium for the lymphatic system. The intake of water aids in maintaining the appropriate level of lymph fluid, which in turn allows for proper functioning of the lymphatic system.

You should drink approximately six to eight 8-oz. glasses of water each day. Soda, coffee, and black tea are not substitutes. All other liquids, including vegetable and fruit juices, should be counted as food, not drink.

It is recommended that you not drink water, or any other fluids other than vegetable or fruit juices, with your meals since water can dilute the digestive juices, reducing your ability to properly digest your meal. (Vegetable and fruit juices contain enzymes that aid in the digestive process.)

Fats

Since one of the lymphatic system's main jobs is to transport fats, the types and amount of fats that are taken in need to be carefully considered. It is important that you reduce the amount of fat in your diet, but it is also important that the fats that you do eat are the ones that are beneficial to your health. It is becoming increasingly obvious that different types of fat have different effects when ingested; yet sorting out which is which can be somewhat confusing. What follows is a basic breakdown of the different types of fat, with recommendations on which to avoid and which to favor.

Saturated Fats should be avoided. They raise LDL cholesterol (the bad kind) and can lead to clogging of the arteries. The lymphatic system must also deal with these fats. There is some evidence that they may increase the risk of certain types of cancer. Saturated fats are found primarily in animal products, including meat, poultry and dairy products, but can also be found in palm and coconut oil, which are commonly used in baked goods.

Monounsaturated Fats should be eaten in moderation. They lower LDL cholesterol levels and may be linked to a reduced incidence of certain cancers. Monounsaturated fats can be found in olive, peanut and canola oils, as well as in a variety of nuts, including cashews and almonds. They can also be found in avocados. Olive, peanut and canola oils are heat resistant, and a good choice for sautéing and baking, making for a healthier circulatory and healthier lymphatic system.

Polyunsaturated Fats, once labeled as good fats, have fallen out of favor. Recent research has linked these fats to increased cancer rates and inflammation. They are high in Omega-6 fatty acids, which are necessary in limited amounts, but only in proportion to Omega-3 fatty acids. The recommended ratio of Omega-6s to Omega-3s is 4 to 1; the current intake in this country is closer to 20 to 1. Polyunsaturated fats can be found in corn, safflower, soybean, sunflower, cottonseed, sesame, walnut, and hazelnut oils. They should not be used in dishes that are heated.

Omega-3 Essential Fatty Acids have recently come into the spotlight as almost "miracle fats." They are being linked to a reduction in heart disease, and are being clinically tested for their role in the treatment of a number of diseases, including some mental disorders. They may also be important in the prevention of some cancers. Unfortunately, Americans have a very low Omega-3 intake. Omega-3 fatty acids can be found in cold-water fish with a high fat content, including salmon, sardines, herring, and mackerel. They can also be found in walnuts and flax seed.

Hydrogenated Fats are those whose molecular structure has been altered through the addition of hydrogen molecules, which creates trans-fatty acids. This process is used to make fats more stable, thus increasing their shelf life, and is widely used in the manufacturing of processed foods. Unfortunately, trans-fatty acids act like saturated fats in the body, and are now being linked to a host of health problems, among them cancer and heart disease. They should be avoided at all cost. They can be found in margarine, vegetable oils, most baked goods, deep-fried foods, and many pre-packaged foods (read labels).

Summary

Most health-care professionals now recommend that total fat intake not fall below 20% nor exceed 30% of total caloric intake. Some recommend fat intakes as low as 10%, especially for people diagnosed with heart disease, although there is little consensus as to whether a diet this low in fat would be healthy for the general population. The fats that are eaten should be primarily monounsaturated fats, with an increase in the amount of Omega-3 fatty acids. Saturated fats and hydrogenated fats should be avoided and polyunsaturated fats should be eaten in moderation. This is especially important for those with or at risk for lymphedema. Being mindful of fats and proteins can make the difference between a congested lymphatic system and one able to manage the lymph volume.

Since the human body tends

to move

in the direction

of its expectations –

plus or minus -

it is important to know

that attitudes of

confidence

and

determination

are no less a part

of the treatment program

than medical science

and technology.

– Norman Cousins

Vitamins-How much is Enough?

Many people have asked my opinion about vitamins to supplement their nutrition. So let's take a look at Balanced Living by Ed Rocks Ph.D. and Handbook for Health by Harold J. Reilly and Ruth Hagy Brod. These two sources of information are written from the Edgar Cayce perspective.

There are thirteen vitamins. Four of these vitamins, A, D, E and K, are fat-soluble and are stored in the body. The other nine are vitamin C and the eight B vitamins. These latter vitamins are water-soluble and are not stored in the body in any appreciable amounts. Some researchers say that you cannot take too many water-soluble vitamins, but there is evidence to show this is not true. For example, when women take excessive amounts of B-6 for menstrual problems they develop severe neurological symptoms. Excesses of Vitamin D (2000 IU) will take calcium from the bones and deposit it in other places, such as the kidneys. When people stopped taking excessive doses these problems disappeared. More is not always better!

In one of the Cayce readings for a health problem he states that, "These (health) disturbances arise from too great a concentrated form of vitamins." He went on to say that all the health problems that this person was experiencing were from excess vitamins. Andrew Weil is a promoter of taking supplements. He would, for example, have you take 5000 mg of Vitamin C each day. In order to receive that in a natural way you would have to eat 166 oranges. Does this sound natural to you? Again, more is not better. Use common sense.

Cayce did say that vitamins are food for the glands and that nature's way is best. The glands in turn supply the energies to the various organs of the body to reproduce themselves. One should eat a large raw salad of lettuce, cabbage, carrots, onions, radishes, peppers, etc as one meal a day. Scraping and grating vegetables and combining these with gelatin will promote even better absorption.

Let's look at what a few of these vitamins will do from a

Cayce perspective. Vitamin A supplies energies to the bone, nerves and brain. Vitamins B and B-1 are suppliers of energy for the white blood cells, controlling the influence of fats and reflexes throughout the body. Vitamin C supplies energies to all the various flexes of the body whether muscular or tendon, heart reaction or kidney contraction and lymph angion peristaltic action. From these few examples we can see how necessary vitamins are to the functioning of our bodies. These vitamins do not come from eating fat laden and starchy foods. "Vegetables will build gray matter faster than meat and sweets!"

In another reading a person asked if they were taking enough vitamins. He replied, "(you are taking)...vitamins to such an extent as to cause the glands to become weakened or fagged by over energizing. Hence we should reduce the quantity." Excessive consumption of vitamins can attack your body just as bacteria do. If the vitamins that enter the system are not put to work in the activities of the body, they affect the plasma of the blood and become destructive to the tissue.

Researchers gave smokers large amounts of beta-carotene, a "known cancer-fighter" to prevent lung cancer. Astonishingly, the incidence of cancer increased in these people by 28%. Why? Perhaps the answer is in this Cayce reading: "This does not mean that it (taking vitamin pills) may be overdone as a preventative or in cases where infection already exists. For, that which may be helpful may also be harmful-if misapplied..." Too much of a good thing can be harmful.

Along with vitamins, there are fifteen major minerals that are essential to good health, such as calcium (a necessary ingredient for lymph movement), magnesium, iodine and selenium. We have established that we need to exercise caution when dealing with supplements. But it seems the more medical information we hear in the daily media and from researchers, the more confusing the information.

First and foremost we need to look at the foods we eat and any other things that find their way into our mouths. If Mother

Nature does its best then let's let her do for our bodies. We can see from very basic information on the function of the immune system how we help our bodies through common sense use of foods and food combining. Supplying complex carbohydrates, raw vegetables and fruit in abundance, and proteins or starches as compliments, will serve to help the body. Just as excess vitamins can hinder, so can excess foods and poor combinations congest the body.

There may be times when a person is run down and needs vitamins and mineral supplements for a short period of time. However, they are not to be taken for long periods of time. Vegetable juicing is a great way to look to Mother Nature for a supplement. I drink 3 oz of vegetable juice made from carrots, celery, raw beet with stalks and red cabbage each weekday. This gives me vitamin C, folates, carotenoids, phytochemicals, etc.

For other supplements, I again look to Mother Nature; I use flax seed oil (Omega 3 with ligians), cod liver oil (vitamin A & D, Omega 3), and wheat germ oil (vitamin E). All these are available at your local health food store. In addition to these, I use Calcios (predigested calcium) and vitamin B complex with iron in raisin juice (available from the Heritage Store, 800-862-2923). Taking only small amounts (a teaspoon a day) and varying the supplements from day to day give the body a nudge rather than overload it. Never take more than two tablespoons of any supplement a week and take a break from any supplement for one week every three to four weeks.

Research by J.R. and Judith R. Casley-Smith, in their book *High Protein Oedemas and the Benzo-Pyrones,* show that without certain vitamins (C and P) present, the intercellular junctions are not tightly knit. This additional space allows micro edemas to occur in tissue. Looking at the body, it consists of one -third solids, and two-thirds liquid. In total, the body consists of 5% blood, 15% connective tissue fluid, 40%-45% intracellular fluid and 30%-35% solids. With the majority of the body being fluid we can readily see how an increase could cause an adverse effect on the lymphatic system. Less material for the lymphatic system (especially a compromised area) and better lymphatic transport depend upon mindfulness of foods, vitamins, and minerals and maintaining a balanced pH.

Vitamins and minerals in natural forms are building blocks for good health. It is important to educate ourselves on the tremendous impact on our well-being that vitamins and minerals have.

SUPPLEMENT SCHEDULE
AFTER FOUR FIVE DAY WEEKS TAKE A WEEK
OFF – REPEAT
Liquids are a teaspoon only or changes are indicated

	Monday	Tuesday
WEEK 1	*Liquid Cod Liver oil *Calcios – half teaspoon *Liquid Vitamin B complex in raisin juice	*Flax oil *Formula "636" – half teaspoon *Iron tablet – one *Glyco-Thymoline – four drops in a bottle of water for the day
WEEK 2	*Flax oil *Liquid Vitamin B complex in raisin juice *Calcios – half teaspoon *Formula "636" – half teaspoon	*Liquid Cod Liver oil *Calcios – half teaspoon *Liquid Vitamin B complex in raisin juice
WEEK 3	*Multi vitamin *Liquid Cod Liver oil *Glyco-Thymoline – four drops in a bottle of water for the day *Iron tablet - one	*Flax oil *Liquid Vitamin B complex in raisin juice *Calcios – half teaspoon *Formula "636" – half teaspoon
WEEK 4	*Wheat germ oil *Calcios – half teaspoon *Liquid Vitamin B complex in raisin juice	*Multi vitamin *Liquid Cod Liver oil *Glyco-Thymoline – four drops in a bottle of water for the day *Iron tablet - one

	Wednesday	Thursday	Friday
WEEK 1	*Wheat germ oil *Calcios – half tea-spoon *Liquid Vitamin B complex in raisin juice	*Multi vitamin *Liquid Cod Liver oil *Glyco-Thymoline – four drops in a bottle of water for the day *Iron tablet - one	*Flax oil *Liquid Vitamin B complex in raisin juice *Calcios – half teaspoon *Formula "636" – half teaspoon
WEEK 2	*Flax oil *Formula "636" – half teaspoon *Iron tablet – one *Glyco-Thymoline – four drops in a bottle of water for the day	*Wheat germ oil *Calcios – half tea-spoon *Liquid Vitamin B complex in raisin juice	*Multi vitamin *Liquid Cod Liver oil *Glyco-Thymoline – four drops in a bottle of water for the day *Iron tablet - one
WEEK 3	*Liquid Cod Liver oil *Calcios – half teaspoon *Liquid Vitamin B complex in raisin juice	*Flax oil *Formula "636" – half teaspoon *Iron tablet – one *Glyco-Thymoline – four drops in a bottle of water for the day	*Wheat germ oil *Calcios – half tea-spoon *Liquid Vitamin B complex in raisin juice
WEEK 4	*Flax oil *Liquid Vitamin B complex in raisin juice *Calcios – half tea-spoon *Formula "636" – half teaspoon	*Liquid Cod Liver oil *Calcios – half teaspoon *Liquid Vitamin B complex in raisin juice	*Flax oil *Formula "636" – half teaspoon *Iron tablet – one *Glyco-Thymoline – four drops in a bottle of water for the day

Each day take the juice of 1/2 freshly squeezed lemon in 1/3 glass of water. Rinse your mouth with water after taking. Do not have any starch within an hour before or after taking the lemon juice.

**".....it is upon Health, not upon ill health
that our sights should be fixed"
- Dr. Roger J. Williams, D.S. & Nutrition**

Obesity – Lymphedema – Lipedema

How do you know if you are obese or just plain overweight? We know that one is considered obese when we exceed by 20% our normal body weight based on sex, age, height and body build. Another way is to look at your body mass index (BMI), with which I am sure many of you are familiar. To calculate your BMI, divide your weight in pounds by your height in inches, squared, and multiply that total by 703. Or, you can go to www.cdc.gov and search obesity, where you will find a BMI chart. Your BMI, of course, is not the last word. If you are a line backer for a professional football team you will not register correctly. It is, however, a good guide for the average person. A person with a BMI of 25 to 30 would be considered overweight; over 30 would be considered obese. A person who is 5'4" tall and weighs 174 pounds is obese. The number one strike against lymphedema is being overweight, and it is important to keep your BMI in the 21, 22 or 23 range. The body is normally composed of 25% fat for the average person.

Having a high BMI is an unfortunate problem not just in our society, but throughout the world. Amazingly, in the past, one of the major causes of death was starvation; now our society, as well as some others, is threatened with the opposite problem. The spread of obesity walks hand in hand with the "fast food industry" as it marches around the world, and therein lies some of the solution. The movie *Super Size Me* provides a glimpse of the starches, fats and sugars that eating a diet of fast food brings to the body; the movie is entertaining, alarming and informative.

Western medicine has therapies to offer for treatment of obesity, some being non-invasive while others put your very life at risk. With the projection of one out of every five health care system dollars being spent on the treatment of obesity, a look at the holistic

perspective is warranted. In the *Physicians Reference Notebook*
is an article by William A McGarey, MD. Dr. McGarey writes in
depth on obesity from the perspective of the Edgar Cayce readings.
The Edgar Cayce readings addressed one hundred and twenty readings regarding obesity, giving such reasons as poor diet, glandular
in-coordination, poor circulation (I imagine poor lymph circulation to be a major factor) and eliminations. The readings give four
major causes of obesity.

The first cause is an "excess of starches in the diet." This
excess of starches in the diet cause poisons in the system. The
poisons in turn "make for a hardening upon the activity of the glandular system as related to the glands of the body" - 1268-2. The
endocrine glands, tissue of the small intestine, and the glandular
tissue that controls the cellular structure unique to reproduction of
specialized tissue apparently are affected by this excess consumption of starches. We see this described in this reading: "there has
been produced in the glands---where the changes take place in the
digestive system, just below the duodenum, that condition wherein
most things turn to sugars, and these increase the avoirdupois of
the system, especially about these portions of the body---the torso
proper." - 5603-1. It appears from this information that overeating
starches is the prime cause of obesity and that this excess of starch,
which turns to sugar, which in turn is stored on the body as fat,
causes abnormalities to occur in the digestive tissues.

The second cause given is the improper or inadequate eliminations of the body. Improvement and balance is needed between the
liver, kidneys, lung, and skin.

The third cause given is glandular imbalance. Although there
are many glandular structures in the body, the primary malfunction
seems to occur in the pineal and adrenals.

The fourth cause given is an unbalance between the sympathetic and parasympathetic divisions of the nervous system. This
imbalance while not primary in cause, however, is mentioned
several times and is part of the process of the body being off center.

It is important for us to remember that the Edgar Cayce readings were given to individuals, and their cause of disease was unique unto them as well as the therapy that was outlined to rebalance the body. With the information given we still can look for repeating information, which indicates a generality, and apply this information to develop a treatment plan.

Dr. McGarey reminds us that it is generally believed that obesity causes other diseases. Perhaps in light of the causes mentioned in Edgar Cayce's Readings we should say that obesity accompanies other diseases caused by these imbalances and the body's attempt to align itself to these malfunctions. Lymphedema is one of those unbalances that may accompany excess weight.

First and foremost we should always remember that the body has the ability to function normally. It is up to us to remove the stumbling blocks that cause the imbalance rather than force the body in one direction or another without addressing the root cause. "Thus, we would administer those activities which would bring a normal reaction through these portions, stimulating them to an activity from the body itself, rather than the body becoming dependent upon supplies that are robbing portions of the system to produce activity in other portions, or the system receiving elements or chemical reactions being applied without arousing the activity of the system itself for a more normal condition." - 1968-3

In the following rational of therapy I will address some therapies that can be instrumental in helping the body to achieve balance. We need to approach any therapy in a persistent and consistent manner, giving the body ample time to adjust. The body can heal in many ways; however, do not jump from one to another - doing a lot of different therapies that will only confuse the body. Allow the body to make slow adjustments to balance. There are many therapies that can be helpful; here I am giving some basic simple ideas.

Rationale of Therapy: The first cause is the eating of excess starches in the diet. These are apparently being turned to sugar by the body and stored. The sugars from starches are causing an addiction that goes even to the cellular level, causing a relentless craving for starch. You can supply sugars to the body without the addiction by simply drinking thirty minutes prior to every meal and at bed time a small juice glass of one third (2oz.) Concord grape juice (preferably organic) and two thirds (4oz.) water. You may not need to do this as outlined if you are only overweight and not obese. In that case you may wish to do it two or three times a week. This will stop the craving for starches. You will need to increase your vegetables and fruits, and follow food-combining rules. Most of all be patient and persistent as the body begins its transition to new balance.

Eating this way will allow the body to have a balanced pH and free calcium available for peristaltic action of the lymph system. Keep moderation in mind and begin this change with one meal a day for several weeks, adding another meal to the day until gradually all of the day's meals are friendly. Slowly work your way up to six days a week. Allow one day to eat whatever you want so as not to feel enslaved by this food idea. After your holiday of foods get yourself back on track so your body's digestive tract will slowly change from turning starches into sugar to digesting a balanced diet, which will in turn lead to a normal body. Keep in mind that a body with excess weight is starved for nutrients from fruits and vegetables. Restricting caloric intake will not be successful in reducing weight. You must change the foods you are ingesting and do moderate exercises; only then will your body automatically lose weight.

The second cause is poor eliminations. We need to improve the work of the liver, kidneys, lungs and skin. Drink 6 - 8 glasses of water a day - water, not tea or coffee - and the flushing of the body will begin. Take a thirty-minute walk each day or, depending on your situation, another aerobic exercise. Exercise is good for kidney function, the blood is pumping, the lymph is moving and the lungs are expelling wastes as you put one foot in front of the other. Breaking a good sweat will allow the skin to expel waste products. Avoid using lotions that will clog the pores of the skin and antiperspirants on the axillary lymph nodes as these may affect your eliminations. Use fifty percent olive oil (4 oz) and peanut oil (4oz.) with a few drops of essential oil of lavender as a food for your skin; this will stimulate the circulation and the lymphatic flow plus provide food for a healthy skin.

The third cause is glandular imbalance. Glandular balance will have to be restored to bring the body into balance. Taking Atomidine was described over and over again as a method to stimulate glands toward normal function. One of the series is as follows: One drop a day in a small glass of water for five days, then rest for five days. Repeat this therapy regimen for a long period of time. Another method is to use the impedance device with atomidine in the solution jar. This device is used to balance the body's energies and with the atomidine apparently comes an enhancement to treatment. In reading 5603-1 the recommendation was to use the device every other day.

To address the imbalance between the sympathetic and parasympathetic divisions of the nervous systems, the use of the violet ray was recommended. This very easy-to-use hand-held device is described in detail in reading 386-1. This device emits static electricity and can be used up and down the spine for no longer than twenty minutes. Another method of balancing the nervous system is to use neuropathic massage strokes down the spine. These strokes are a circular stroke starting at the cervical vertebra and working down the spine. The circular stroke is done at each vertebra location at approximately one inch off the spine. Another method that I have used is with a small handheld vibrator equipped with the cup end. Staying about one inch off the spine, you go slowly up and down each side of the spine. Using this for twenty minutes is ideal. If you are fortunate enough to have a practicing osteopath in your area you could have osteopathic adjustments to the spine. As many as twenty-eight treatments are recommended for some individuals. The purpose of all these treatments is to give the spine the ability to send out better nerve impulse, in turn giving the body optimal function and regulation of the lymphatic drainage.

Attitude is another important aspect of one's therapy. As we go through life we are spending ourselves, so to speak. It is important that we spend our lives in a direction we are interested in and in a way that makes the world a better place for all of us. This gives purpose to our life.

Reading this information and gaining knowledge will be worthless unless action is taken. We must realize that the body will need action and time to find a new balance point. A dysfunctional body is replacing itself through cellular renewal in a dysfunctional way. It will need time as the malfunctioning process is slowly eliminated. You must be persistent and patient. Remember that the body has the ability to function normally.

In "Lymphedema, Diagnosis and Therapy," by Horst Weissleder and Christian Schuchhardt, the typical lipedema patient is a woman with normal hands, feet, and upper limbs. With most cases the lower limbs have an impairment of excess fatty tissue. Treatment may be plastic surgery or liposuction to relieve this painful impairment.

What is happening when the fat becomes deposited in an abnormal amount on certain areas of the body? Dr. McGarey refers to this as "Disproportion of Body Parts." He is saying that faulty eliminations are the principal etiological agent of fat being deposited in areas of the body that are not proportional to the rest of the body. The Cayce readings say that all diseases through history are the same, only the names have changed over time. I believe what is being described in the following reading is Lipedema.

An extract from the readings:
"......eliminations are those that cause the disorders in the lower portions of the system, feet, ankles, and limbs, as well as those that produce a tendency for portions of the body, especially, to be out of proportion to the body as a whole.

The conditions...may be aided the most were the body to be more mindful of the diet; not as an extremist, no --- but as one that would have the corrections make in the general eliminating system.

. . . this would be . . . an outline for the corrections of the physical conditions, that may later produce hindrances in the general physical health of the body."

We would begin first with colonic irrigations---one every ten days until four or five are taken, which will overcome this tendency of constipation through the system.

We would, also, at least twice a week, have sweat cabinet baths, with a thorough rubdown afterwards with any of the eliminates or prepare as this: Take Russian white oil, one pint; alcohol, one pint; witch hazel, one-half pint. Mix these together and massage the body with same following the baths, see? Well to occasionally leave off the oil rub and use the salt glow (that is, rub the body with salt)." - 2096-1

Foods are addressed as we continue on in reading 2096-1. "For the matter of diet, we would use citrus fruits, or stewed fruits, or the whole dried or dried cereal. Do not combine same! That is, when one is used do not use the other - but these may be changed or altered, as this: The juice of two or three oranges, or one grapefruit, with dried toast following, with either Ovaltine or a cereal drink. Little coffee, little milk, or little tea may be taken. For the noon meals, preferably green vegetables - with any of the oil dressings. All green vegetables, see?' Of evenings, we would take fish, honey (in the honeycomb) - not too much, cooked vegetables, no potatoes of any character; no tuberous roots of any character, but any of the green vegetables cooked, or of the dried vegetables that grow above the ground - cooked. Little ice cream or none. Little or no butter. Buttermilk may be taken occasionally, but be mindful that it is not taken with too many of the vegetables."

We can readily see that the food selected is taking the strain off the digestive system. Large green salads are very alkalizing to the body and are nerve building. The cooked vegetables (I would recommend steamed) are much easier to digest, especially as we become sedentary during the evening hours. This will help the pH balance and provide calcium for the lymph system's smooth muscle to move the lymph. The reading goes on to say that this will make for normal forces in the body. All of us have our strengths and weaknesses; we need to bolster our weaknesses if we want health. Management through the foods we eat can lead us to lasting health.

All of the therapy tools mentioned in this information are available through the Heritage Store in Virginia Beach, Virginia, phone 1-800-862-2923 or www.caycecures.com.

Concord Grape Juice

Many individuals in our society struggle with the constant problem of being overweight, and since excess weight has a negative impact on lymphedema, we should look at a very simple and interesting way of controlling weight from the Edgar Cayce readings. This method of losing weight is called the "Grape Juice Way."

It has become clear that eating excess starch is the number one cause of being overweight. The sugars that come from starches are addictive, even on the cellular level. This addiction to starches can be offset by substituting a sugar that does not itself cause addiction. This allows the person to stop the cravings, and eat a more healthful diet composed of vegetables and fruits, complemented by whole grains or small amounts of light protein.

The "Grape Juice Way" goes like this: thirty minutes before each meal and at bedtime drink 2 oz. of Concord Grape Juice with 4 oz. of water. This will supply sugar to the body without creating an addiction and will allow better body functioning. You will, of course, also need to make a decision not to continue eating the excess starch and to increase the amount of vegetables and fruits in your meals.

Let's look at some of the Cayce readings to gain more insight into this idea. In the following reading a female that is forty-eight years old is being warned not to become overweight. "We would also indicate that there should be more regular intervals of taking the grape juice systematically as has been indicated. Not that the body is too heavy, but just don't get too heavy for the bettered conditions of heart, lungs, liver and kidneys" 1100-38. The reading goes on to tell the person to take the grape juice for a month to six weeks, stop for 2 to 3 weeks and then to take it again. The reading also warns of attitude; when disturbing mental relationships occur, not to be upset. In another reading it states the grape juice will reduce the desire for foods that produce flesh. This method reduces not only the desire for excess starches; it also reduces the desire for excess sweets. We can all relate to this when we approach any holiday season. The readings say that Concord grape juice will aid the glands related to digestion, control the appetite, and aid in eliminations. They also warned of being patient with weight loss. As the BMI comes down to the 21 - 23 range we would use the grape juice a few days a week.

Even my favorite local market tells us to "strive for five" servings of vegetables and fruit each day. Many weight loss groups don't count vegetables, and the Cayce readings tell us to make them between 60-80% of our diet for good reason. Vegetables contain the building blocks for the construction of our bodies and don't produce excess flesh. Add moderate exercise, and a prayerful attitude, and you have the formula for good health along with improving peristaltic action of the lymph system. With more and more articles mentioning how weight is a factor with lymphedema, it is important to keep our body mass index in the 21 – 23 range, which will help lymph flow. By focusing on eating all the green foods to keep our bodies alkaline, exercising, receiving MLD treatments, and using compression, you will be better able to manage your lymphedema, and with less maintenance.

> **"Where the willingness is great,**
> **the difficulties cannot be great"**
> **-Niccolo Mechiavelli**

Food Combining

In the treatment of your lymphedema, the acid-alkaline balance is a critical ingredient. Proper food combining helps control the number of acids being introduced into the body at any one time, which in turn allows the acid-alkaline balance of the blood to remain relatively stable. Keeping the blood from becoming too acidic means that more free calcium is available in the body, since it is not used to buffer the high blood acidity. This calcium is then available for the peristaltic motion of the lymphatic vessels, which in turn leads to a healthier lymphatic system.

Learning how to combine proteins, fats, and starches will help your digestive system as well. It may seem complicated at first, but once you understand the **Three Simple Rules,** it becomes habit:

- **Avoid protein with starch**
- **Avoid starch with starch**
- **Avoid citrus with starch**

In other words:

- Proteins combine with starchless vegetables.
- Starches combine with starchless vegetables and fats.
- Acidic fruits combine with each other, and with starchless vegetables, and with protein fats.
- Sub-acidic fruits combine with each other.
- Sweet fruits combine with each other.
- Melon should be eaten alone.
- Sweeteners should be eaten with whole grains.
- All dairy products, with the exception of yogurt, should be avoided by adults.

The food-combining information that begins on page 47 lists the different categories of foods and identifies what can be combined with what.

Friendly Food Guidelines

To create the best acid-alkaline balance, build your meals around a variety of vegetables and fruits (60-80% of what you eat) with an emphasis on those vegetables that grow above the ground (starchless), rather than below. Prepare these vegetables separately to preserve their taste, steaming them (using a stainless steel steamer) in a granite or enameled pan or cooking them in patapar paper (available at cooking stores). You can also use a stainless steel pressure cooker or bake in the oven. When preparing your meals, do not use aluminum cooking utensils or accessories as aluminum has a negative effect on the lymphatic system.

The rest of your meal (20-40%) should be made up of whole grains, starch vegetables, proteins, and fats. Starches should be limited to one per meal. Use a variety of whole grains, including brown rice, whole wheat couscous, and whole grain breads. Whole grain pasta should be eaten sparingly; choose brown rice or corn pastas instead, which are much lighter. Some people have reported an increase in their lymphedema after consuming whole-wheat foods; if you find this to be the case, eliminate them from your diet. When eating animal protein, choose lighter proteins such as lamb, fish or fowl that have been baked or broiled. Protein servings should not exceed 3.5 ounces and should be about the size of the palm of your hand and approximately of the same thickness.

Drink 3-4 ounces of vegetable juice five days a week, preferably at lunchtime with a large salad. The nutrients and enzymes found in vegetable juices help create the building blocks for a healthy lymphatic system. Carrots, beets, celery, and a small wedge of red cabbage are all good juicing vegetables. For convenience, the juice can be prepared ahead of time and be kept in the refrigerator for up to two days. (See juice recipe, pg. 63)

Create a calm and relaxing environment when you eat, making meals an enjoyable and social experience for yourself and your family. Avoid eating when angry, excited, or very tired.

Drink six to eight glasses of water daily to keep your body hydrated and to flush out toxins. Do not drink water with meals as it can dilute the digestive juices. To keep track of your water intake during each day, you may want to fill two 32-ounce containers with water in the morning, and drink from those. Consider using a reverse osmosis water filtration system or other filtration system (Brita, for example) to remove chloride, bacteria, etc.

Use salt sparingly and only use sea salt that has been sun dried. Commercial salt has been heat processed and bleached with chemicals and aluminum stearate may have been added to prevent clumping. Choose a baking powder without aluminum as an ingredient for your baking needs. Aluminum has a negative effect on the lymphatic system.

Use oils high in monounsaturated fats. These oils include olive, canola, and peanut; whenever possible, purchase cold-pressed organic oils and use these oils for sautéing and baking.

Avoid fried foods, heavily spiced foods, candy, cake, pastries, sugar-coated cereals, processed foods, pork (including bacon), white flour, white sugar, white bread, white potatoes, and white pastas, carbonated beverages, prepared frozen foods, alcohol and tobacco, coffee and tea, red meat, and dairy products (except for plain yogurt). These foods are difficult to digest, may be empty in nutrients, contain saturated fats, and dehydrate and/or are acidic in nature, causing a disruption in the body's metabolism and chemical balance, leading to acidity, which may further congest the lymphatic system.

If you take supplements, do so only from a natural source and only in moderation as more is not better and toxic levels may accumulate in the body.

Plain yogurt is an active cleanser to the intestinal system and to the colon. A cleaner colon will lead to a healthier lymphatic system. Yogurt has predigested fat, sugar, and protein which lightens the work load on the body since it does not have to produce more digestive enzymes.

Friendly Food Combining

STARCHLESS VEGETABLES

Starchless vegetables, along with fruits, should make up 60-80% of your total intake. Starchless vegetables should be eaten with one choice only of fat, starch, animal protein, protein fat or protein starch.

Artichoke
Asparagus
Bamboo shoot
Bell peppers
Beet tops
Bok choy
Broccoli
Brussel Sprouts
Cabbage-red
Cabbage-green
Carrots
Cauliflower
Celery
Chard
Chive
Collard greens
Cucumber
Dandelion greens
Eggplant
Endive
Escarole

Garlic
Green beans
Kale
Leeks
Lettuce (leafy)
Mushrooms
Mustard greens
Okra
Onions
Parsley
Peas
Radishes
Spinach
Sprouts
Summer squash
Swiss chard
Turnip tops
Watercress
Yellow beans
Zucchini

PROTEIN STARCH
EAT WITH STARCHLESS VEGETABLES

Beans (dry)   Peas (dry)
Soy beans (soy bean products)   Lentils

ANIMAL PROTEIN
EAT WITH STARCHLESS VEGETABLES

Beef (avoid)   Fish   Pork (avoid)   Seafood
Eggs (whole)   Lamb   Poultry

PROTEIN FAT
EAT WITH STARCHLESS VEGETABLES OR FRUIT

Avocado   Kefir Cheese
Seeds   Olives
Nuts (except chestnut and peanut)   Soy cheese
Plain low fat yogurt
Dairy – avoid with the exception of yogurt

MILD STARCH VEGETABLES
EAT WITH STARCHLESS VEGETABLES; FATS

Beets   Salsify
Parsnips   Turnips
Rutabaga

HIGH-STARCH FOODS
EAT WITH STARCHLESS VEGETABLES OR FAT

Bread - whole grain only   Peanuts- eat in moderation
Chestnuts   Sweet Potato w/skin
Corn-eat in moderation   (eat sparingly)
Crackers - whole grain   Pumpkin
Dry cereals -   Rice (brown)
   add water or eat alone   Squash (winter)
Grains –whole grains   Popcorn (eat sparingly)
Jerusalem artichoke   Yams/Sweet potatoes
Lima beans
Pastas - avoid white; choose corn, brown rice
   or whole wheat pastas - eat sparingly

FATS
EAT WITH PROTEIN FAT, STARCHES, AND STARCHLESS VEGETABLES

Butter (sparingly)
Margarine (avoid)

Cream (sparingly)
Oils (See pg. 25-26 for additional information.)

FRUITS, ACID
EAT ALONE OR WITH EACH OTHER, OR COMBINE WITH PROTEIN FAT OR STARCHLESS VEGETABLE

Apples (sour)*
Cherries (sour)
Cranberry
Currant
Gooseberry
Grapefruit
Grapes(sour)
Kumquat
Lemon
• Lime

Loganberry
Orange
Pineapple
Plums (sour)
Pomegranate
Strawberry
Tangelo
Tangerine
Tomato*

*tomatoes should not be eaten with peaches
*raw apples should always be eaten alone

FRUIT, SWEET
EAT ALONE OR WITH EACH OTHER

Dried*		Fresh
Apple*	Pears	Bananas*
Apricot	Peaches	Grapes (sweet)
Banana*	Pineapple	Persimmon
Dates	Prune	
Figs	Raisins	

*apples and bananas should not be combined with other fruits or each other
*all dried fruits should be unsulfured and reconstituted before eating

FRUIT, SUB-ACID
EAT ALONE OR WITH EACH OTHER

Apples (sweet)*
Apricot
Blackberry
Blueberry
Boysenberry
Cherries (sweet)
Elderberry
Figs (fresh)
Guava
Huckleberry

Kiwi
Mango
Mulberry
Nectarine
Papaya
Peach*
Pear
Plum (sweet)
Raspberry

*peaches should not be eaten with tomatoes
*apples should always be eaten alone

MELONS
EAT EACH ALONE

Cantaloupe
Honeydew

Muskmelon
Watermelon

SWEETENERS
EAT ALONE OR WITH WHOLE GRAINS

All Sugar (avoid)
Carob
Honey

Malt
Maple Syrup
Molasses

**"The great end of life is
not knowledge, but action."
- Thomas Henry Huxley**

Friendly Food Planning

The following three-day menu sample of "friendly food" recommendations is designed to help you begin changing your eating habits to better manage lymphedema. Following these recommendations will not result in feelings of deprivation, but will leave you feeling that you have made wise choices which will promote optimal health. This sample menu should help you to begin to understand which foods to avoid and which to emphasize. Be mindful of food combinations to lessen the acid effect on the body; it is not so much the effect of one single food as it is the combinations of acids that cause disruption to the body.

Changing your eating habits can feel like an overwhelming task, but you can make it seem less so by introducing these changes slowly. Begin by eating your new "friendly" food way one day a week for several weeks, then two days, and so on until you have only one day each week of relaxed food considerations. As you change your lifestyle, you'll see a difference in how you feel, which will help you continue your quest for a healthier lymphatic system.

Day One

Breakfast

Begin with a glass of tepid water upon rising to clarify the intestinal system. Make buckwheat, corn (blue corn meal is delicious) or whole-wheat pancakes or waffles from scratch, using honey as a sweetener, and water as the liquid for the batter. A small amount of honey or 'B' grade maple syrup can be used as a topping (See sample recipe). Remember to use a "friendly" oil in your batter. Save the fruit you may wish to use as a topping for your mid-morning break (this will allow for better food combining). Cook in a cast iron pan, using a small amount of olive or canola or peanut oil to prevent sticking.

Snack Time

Fresh or dried unsulfured fruits or a small glass of organic fruit juice.

Lunch

A large raw salad made from fresh green vegetables, including green leafy lettuce, green or red cabbage, celery, spinach, tomatoes (vine ripe when available), onions, radish, leeks, and carrots. Use salad dressing sparingly. Drink your vegetable juice with your salad. A slice of whole wheat (sprouted wheat) or oat or corn (yellow or blue) bread with a small amount of butter would complement the salad nicely.

Or you could substitute a large fruit salad, using fresh, frozen and/or canned fruit. If you do choose the fruit, do not have bread with it, as this would be combining a starch with fruit, which you want to avoid.

Snack Time

A small container of plain yogurt mixed with fresh, frozen or canned fruit.

Dinner

Two or three large portions of starchless vegetables, prepared separately for better taste, and either:

One starch: a baked sweet potato, brown rice, wild rice, or whole grain couscous. Remember the portion percentages (pg. 45).

OR

A piece of lamb, fish or fowl, either baked or broiled (not breaded and fried), the size and thickness of your palm.

Snack Time

It is best to avoid eating at night, but if you can't, *keep it small.* Try a small bowl of organic cereal (eat dry or with water) or a piece of fruit. Do not add soy milk or milk to the cereal, as this would be combining a starch with a protein.

Day Two

Breakfast

A glass of tepid water upon rising to clarify the intestinal system. Old fashioned oatmeal (avoid quick oats), prepared in either a granite or enameled pan. Add maple syrup or honey and/or raw almonds.

Snack Time

Celery or cucumber with natural peanut butter (no added sugar or hydrogenated oils).

Lunch

A cup of homemade soup (commercial soups have a high salt content, which encourages fluid retention). Lentil soup would be a good choice, with a salad or non-starch vegetables. (Since lentils are a starch, another starch would not be added.)

Snack Time

Fresh vegetables or raw almonds.

Dinner

Two or three starchless vegetables or a large quantity of one.

A dish of your choice made from tofu or tempeh. Both of these are soy products and should be considered as meat substitutes. Treat in quantity as you would an animal protein (as large as your palm and no thicker).

No starch should be introduced with the meal.

Snack Time

If necessary, perhaps plain yogurt with fruit.

Day Three

Breakfast

A glass of water upon rising to clarify the intestinal system. Coddled or soft-boiled eggs or an omelet with fresh vegetables.

Snack Time

Soy nuts, figs, prunes or chopped dates or a piece of whole grain bread with a small amount of butter (treat butter as a seasoning).

Lunch

A leftover from the previous evening's meal and a salad.

Snack Time

A few whole grain crackers (without hydrogenated oil) or flat breads or seeds.

Dinner

Prepare any two vegetables, such as cauliflower and kale, and build a meal around them.

There are many low-fat cookbooks that have great recipes. Look for dishes that are not fat and protein laden, or take old recipes and change them to make them friendlier to the body. Don't be afraid to experiment and keep in mind food combining.

Remember the Three Simple Rules:

- **Avoid protein with starch**
- **Avoid starch with starch**
- **Avoid citrus with starch**

Sample Recipes

Pancakes or waffles

You may make a pancake or waffle by a simple and friendly recipe:

In a mixing bowl add:

1 cup of any whole grain flour (vary the grain choice each time): whole wheat, yellow or blue corn, buckwheat, brown rice or rye. Rye works best as a waffle.
Ring of honey (squeeze out honey making a ring or approximately a teaspoon)
1 Teaspoon (heaping) of non-aluminum baking powder
1 Teaspoon of olive, peanut or canola oil
1 egg yolk (discard the white)
Water as needed for the desired consistency

Heat a cast-iron skillet on medium heat, lightly oiled to prevent sticking, and ladle in the batter. Brown as you would like your pancake. Or use a waffle iron lightly oiled if you prefer. You may use honey or maple syrup (B grade) as a topping.

Scrambled eggs

You can spice up scrambled eggs with sautéed peppers (all colors), onions, garlic or other vegetables. Adding a whole grain toast is acceptable, however, do not add a citrus juice. Instead choose apple or grape juice to avoid acid combinations.

Dry cereal

If you are choosing a dry cereal, choose one that is fruit juice sweetened and made from one grain if possible. Avoid acidic animal milk on the cereal; instead make your own almond milk. Simply add 1/3 cup of raw almonds to a cup of water in your blender (you may wish to place the blender in the refrigerator the night before to soften the almonds and chill the water).

If desired, add a small amount of honey or a date and a teaspoon of vanilla extract for sweetness and flavor. Blend until you have almond milk. By making your own almond milk you can avoid the sugar that is in commercial brands.

Lamb, Fish or Fowl

With either of these lighter proteins it is a simple and quick meal. Simply spray with olive oil, rub in the spices of your choice, place on a rack and bake at 25 to 30 minutes at 375 degrees. I use this method for lamb chops, fish filets, or fowl. Wash and chop your three vegetables and place in three steamers; with the oven preheated you can start your entire meal at once and it will be ready in 30 minutes. If you are steaming collard greens or kale you could add sautéed onions, peppers of various colors and garlic to enhance the greens, and mist on some olive oil. A small portion of salad is fine with the evening meal. There are no complicated recipes to follow that can be time consuming and in many cases are suspect in nourishing the body.

Changing a Recipe

Let's look at a poor food combining recipe for salmon cakes:

One 15 oz. can of salmon (protein – acid)
    ½ cup of bread crumbs (starch – acid)
    Two tablespoons of vegetable oil (fat)
    Two whole eggs (yolk – alkaline, white is protein – acid)
    Sprinkle with paprika (basically for color)

This recipe was suggested to be served over rice (starch – acid).

Remember that we are avoiding starch with protein. We are avoiding acid combinations to conserve the free calcium and avoid the body from having to go to the body's skeleton bank to withdraw calcium.

Let's make it friendly:

One 15 oz. can of salmon rinsed to remove any excess salt (protein – acid)

One yellow or green summer squash, shredded (starchless vegetable – alkaline)

Two egg yolks (alkaline reacting)

Serve with three steamed starchless vegetables (alkaline).

Bake on a rack for 25 - 30 minutes, season with a small amount of Thousand Island dressing or deli mustard of your choice. Complete the meal with a small portion of salad to keep the 60-80% vegetable balance.

Green pizza

As we know, most pizzas are made with white refined flour, which we should avoid. In search of an easy way to make a meal I decided to use whole wheat pita breads. I cut them flat ways so that I can keep less starch with my meal. The two pita breads now become four thin pitas to make up my meal.

Let's continue:

Two whole wheat pitas cut flat ways.

Package of fresh baby spinach blanched.

One 15 oz. can of asparagus (or fresh steamed) or a package of frozen broccoli steamed.

Medium sized onion sautéed with a small amount of water or olive oil seasoned with rubbed sage or spices of your choice.

Slice of fresh tomato slightly blanched.

Arrange the four sliced pitas on a pizza stone, divide up the blanched and drained spinach over the pitas, follow this with the asparagus or broccoli, top these two with the sautéed onion and lastly the slice of tomato. Place in the oven for 12 minutes at 425 degrees. Serve immediately with two steamed vegetables of your choice. You may sprinkle some dried Romano or Parmesan or feta cheese for flavor; use it as a seasoning for taste. We don't have to be perfect, however, we must be mindful.

Dessert

I plan to make an apple pie today. The crust recipe is calling for 2-1/4 cups of all purpose flour; I will immediately change to whole wheat pastry flour or a combination of whole and pastry for a complex carbohydrate rather than a simple carbohydrate. The recipe calls for vegetable shortening which I discover has fully hydrogenated and partially hydrogenated soybean and cottonseed oil. These are comprised of an unnatural molecule. I will use oil in place of the shortening.

> One cup plus a quarter of whole wheat flour
> One cup of whole wheat pastry flour
> Half teaspoon of salt
> Half cup of canola oil
> Half cup of cold water

Chill the dough before working it into the size you need to match your pie plate. The dough may try to crack as you work it to size; don't be discouraged, simply patch it as necessary. The patch will not detract from the taste.

You may find many whole wheat pie crust recipes on the Internet or in your favorite cookbook.

The apples I precook in a small amount of butter and cinnamon and do not add the sugar as called for in the recipe. Apples are sweet themselves and we do not need to add more sugar calories. If you insist on using sugar, use beet sugar if possible and cut the amount in half.

If you have decided to make a cake, again drop the sugar, or cut it in half or a third and use beet in place of cane if possible. Use whole wheat flour or whole wheat pastry flour instead of the all purpose flour. Allow the sweet to come from the frosting, which you have cut back on sugar. Do not have ice cream and cake together; choose one. These small changes are going to be in your favor through less work for the body in compensating for acids. It will also help the compromised area of the lymphatic system by lessening its workload. Begin to experiment with recipes and make them friendlier to yourself. Apply this same idea if you are making cookies for a sweet.

This is a simple method of cooking and is friendlier chemistry to the body. When looking at a recipe keep the "three simple rules" in mind as you change to a friendlier dish. You may change any recipe, though some are hard to save, by following the "Three Simple Rules." Stick to the basics of buffering acids - it doesn't have to be absolutely perfect to make the meal friendly to the body.

If you're having your family for a holiday dinner, make your meal in the traditional fashion to make your family feel welcome. They will enjoy the tradition of a Thanksgiving meal, for example, or other traditional family meal. The next day, go back to being friendly with your foods so as not to overwhelm the compromised area of the lymphatic system. You are looking to follow food combining rules for six days of meals each week.

Always do a variety of foods.

Food Combining Chart

Lines connect the catagories that can be eaten together

Protein Fat

Avocado
Kefir Cheese
Nuts (except chestnut
    and peanut)
Dairy - Avoid all with the
exception of yogurt
Soy Cheese
Yogurt (low fat)
Seeds
Olives

Mild Starch

Beets	Salsify
Parsnips	Turnips
Rutabega	

High Starch

Bread+	*Pasta**
Cereal+	*Peanuts, Raw**
Chestnuts	*Popcorn**
Corn	*Potato* (w/skin)*
Crackers+	Pumpkin
Grains+	Rice (Brown)
Jerusalem	Squash
Artichoke	(winter)
Lima Beans	Yams (w/skin)

+ Whole single grain
products only

Starchless Vegetables

Artichoke	Escarole
Asparagus	Garlic
Bamboo	Green Beans
Shoots	Kale
Bell Peppers	Leeks
Beet Tops	Lettuce (leafy)
Bok Choy	Mushrooms
Broccoli	Mustard Greens
Brussel	Okra
Sprouts	Onions
Cabbage	Parsley
Carrots	Peas
Cauliflower	Radishes
Celery	Spinach
Chard	Sprouts
Chives	Squash
Collard	(summer)
Greens	Swiss Chard
Cucumber	Turnip Tops
Dandelion	Watercress
Eggplant	Yellow Beans
Endive	Zucchini

Starchless Vegetables

Artichoke	Escarole
Asparagus	Garlic
Bamboo	Green Beans
Shoots	Kale
Bell Peppers	Leeks
Beet Tops	Lettuce (leafy)
Bok Choy	Mushrooms
Broccoli	Mustard Greens
Brussel	Okra
Sprouts	Onions
Cabbage	Parsley
Carrots	Peas
Cauliflower	Radishes
Celery	Spinach
Chard	Sprouts
Chives	Squash
Collard	(summer)
Greens	Swiss Chard
Cucumber	Turnip Tops
Dandelion	Watercress
Eggplant	Yellow Beans
Endive	Zucchini

Fats

*Butter**	*Cream**
Margarine (avoid)	Oils

Animal Protein

Beef (avoid)	Pork (avoid)
Eggs (whole)	Poultry
Fish	Seafood
Lamb	

Protein Starch

Beans, Dry
Peas, Dry
Soy Beans
All Soy Products
Lentils

Protein Fat

Avocado
Kefir Cheese
Nuts (except chestnut
    and peanut)
Dairy - Avoid all with the
exception of yogurt
Soy Cheese
Yogurt (low fat)
Seeds
Olives

choose
one
protein
per meal

60

Fruits, Acid		Fruits, Sub-acid	
Fruits, Acid (Eat alone or with each other, or combine with protein fat or non-starch vegetable)		**Fruits, Sub-acid** (Eat alone or combine with each other)	
Apples (sour)*	Loganberry	Apples (sweet)*	Kiwi
Cherries (sour)	Orange	Apricot	Mango
Cranberry	Pineapple	Blackberry	Mulberry
Currant	Plums (sour)	Blueberry	Nectarine
Gooseberry	Pomegranate	Boysenberry	Papaya
Grapefruit	Strawberry	Cherries (sweet)	Peach*
Grapes (sour)	Tangelo	Elderberry	Pear
Kumquat	Tangerine	Figs, Fresh	Plum
Lemon	Tomato*	Guava	(sweet)
Lime		Huckleberry	Raspberry

Fruits, Sweet
(Eat alone or combine with each other)

Dried*	Dates	Pineapple	**Fresh***	Banana
Apple*	Fig	Prune		Grapes
Apricot	Pear	Raisins		Persimmon
Banana	Peach*			

Melons
(Eat each alone)

Cantaloupe	Muskmelon
Honeydew	Watermelon

Sweeteners
(Eat alone or with whole grains)

All Sugar	Honey
(avoid)	Malt
Carob	Molasses
Maple syrup	

NOTES

Foods in italics should be eaten sparingly.
Tomatoes should never be eaten with peaches.
Fruits within each category can be combined with each other.
Raw bananas and raw apples should not be combined with other foods or with each other.
All dried fruits should be unsulfured.
All dried fruits should be reconstituted before eating.
Of your total nutritional intake, 60-80% should consist of fruits and vegetables.

The Road To Success
is Always Under Construction
– Lily Tomlin

Helpful Hints

To insure your water intake, fill two 32 ounce containers with water and empty by the day's end.

If you've been accustomed to eating large amounts of starches, such as crackers, pasta, and bread, you may find yourself craving them. To help the body adjust and to offset this craving, have a glass of 2 oz. organic Concord grape juice and 4 oz. of water 30 minutes prior to each meal and prior to bedtime. (See Concord Grape Juice.)

Having lighter meals and eating more often will allow the body to assimilate the food and use it rather than having to store a large influx of food taken at one time.

Once a week, have an all-citrus fruit breakfast including grapefruit, oranges or pineapple and the juices of the same. Do not combine starches with your citrus fruit breakfast. Each day take the juice of 1/2 freshly squeezed lemon in 1/3 glass of water. Rinse your mouth with water after taking. Do not have any starch within an hour before or after taking the lemon juice. Keeping with food combining rules.

Eat whole eggs as a meal no more than three times a week (eat the whole egg rather than just the whites, which are acidic protein and hard to digest) or eat only the yolk, which is alkaline reacting.

• When eating out, choose carefully from the menu to avoid any fried, heavily spiced or dairy-laden dishes. Choose dishes that are baked or broiled. While you will not always be able to avoid all fats and dairy, you can make the best choices possible for your lymphatic system. Don't be afraid to ask the server for special considerations - ask for your salad dressing on the side and use it sparingly, ask for baked potatoes (eat the skin and a small portion of the starchy center, discard the remainder) with the butter on the side and use it as a seasoning; enjoy the taste without taking in large quantities of saturated fat. Always bear in mind the burden to your lymphatic system; be friendly to yourself.

Beware of dry cereals which have various blends of grains and of soy products composed of soy mixed with rice (some varieties of tempeh). These products combine starch with starch and should be avoided. Read labels! Seek single grains!

We all eat sweets, however it is best to avoid too many. Take only enough to sufficiently provide vitality. Choose your sweets from foods such as raisins, dates, maple syrup or honey. Avoid the sugar and starch combinations found in baked goods. Ice cream is a better choice than cakes, pies, donuts, or pastries.

Vegetable juicers are available at most stores that sell small appliances. The most moderately priced vegetable juicers will suffice to make vegetable juice. A recommended juice recipe is as follows:

> 4 large carrots, tops removed
> 1 large stalk of celery, top and leaves removed
> 1/2 small fresh beet, stalk and greens included
> small wedge of red cabbage

Wash vegetables in sink of cold water, removing all undesirable portions. Process through juicer. This recipe should make approximately four servings of juice, which will keep for two days in the refrigerator. The amount of vegetables used can be adjusted for different quantities of juice and to your taste, or you can freeze any excess juice. Drink 3-4 ounces per day, preferably at lunchtime with your salad. Vegetable juice should be treated as a supplement as well as a food, and should not be consumed in quantities greater than listed above.

Holistic Health Recommendations

A natural homeopathic remedy, **Cimex Lectularius**, is recommended for phlebitis (inflammation of a vein) and edema (swelling due to lymph accumulation of water retention); it works by acting on the parasympathetic and sympathetic systems.

The parasympathetic and sympathetic systems work in opposition to each other; one inhibits bodily functions and the other excites. Each system releases different neurotransmitters and has different neurotransmitter receptors in its affected tissues. Balancing the two systems is a major component of good health.

The parasympathetic system is active when the body is at rest and non-threatened. It regulates the housekeeping functions of the body, including digestion and elimination and decreases the demands placed on the heart and circulatory system.

The sympathetic system, on the other hand, is often   referred to as the "fight or flight" system because it prepares the body to deal with stressful situations that will affect the body's homeostasis. Sympathetic conditions increase heart rate, blood pressure, blood sugar levels and dilate the bronchioles of the lungs. The smooth muscle in the walls of the blood arteries and the lymphatic ducts are also affected.

Cimex Lectularius can be used to help balance these two divisions of the autonomic nervous systems, resulting in a stimulation of lymph flow. It is described as that which *takes the place* of atropine. Atropine is an alkaloid from Atropa Belladonna and Datura Stramonium plants. It is related to other drugs such as scopolamine and hyoscyamine. Atropine has a similar action of blocking parasympathetic stimuli by raising the threshold of response of effector cells to acetylcholine. This homeopathic remedy may help primary lymphedema.

Cimex Lectularius is available through health stores.

Mullein tea aids in reducing the tendencies for the accumulation of lymph through the abdomen and the limbs. This will *stimulate* the lymphatic system. Sip 1/3 cup of weak mullein tea throughout the day. Do not use with other diuretic medications.

Watermelon seed tea *stimulates* elimination through kidney lymphatics. Drink 8 oz. each day. Use with caution if you have weak digestion, anemia, or uncontrolled urination. Do not use with other diuretic medications. (Available through health stores).

Senna tea has a drying effect upon the lymph. Drink a tea cup full once or twice a day, carefully following the directions on the package. Do not use for long periods of time as senna has a laxative effect and your body may develop a dependence, and do not use with any other diuretic medications. Senna may irritate the digestive tract, cause bloody diarrhea, vomiting or dehydration. Discontinue if any of these symptoms occur.

Spinal subluxations are incomplete dislocations of spinal vertebrae, which could affect edema. Your chiropractor can evaluate whether or not you have a spinal subluxation that may be impinging upon a nerve and affecting your health.

Vitamins A, B complex, C, D, E, and P are important to a healthy circulatory and lymphatic system, taken in quantities that do not upset the system. While it is always preferable to get your nutrients from food, sometimes supplementation can be beneficial. Food sources of these vitamins include: wheat germ oil in liquid form for vitamin E - 2 tablespoons a week recommended. Emphasizing the yellow food group (egg yolks, yellow summer squash, peaches, etc.), brewer's yeast and blackstrap molasses provide vitamin B complex. Carrot juice is a good source of beta-carotene, which is transformed into vitamin A in the body. Cod liver oil, one teaspoon daily, is one of the best sources of vitamin D and is high in vitamin A as well. Vegetable juice is a good source of vitamin C, and citrus fruits provide both vitamin C and P. (Refer to the supplement schedule on page 32.)

Colonic irrigation is the most thorough and effective method of cleaning the whole length of the colon. If a professional is unavailable to administer the colonic it may be done with a three-stage enema as follows:

Purchase an enema kit from your local medical supply store or pharmacy.

First bag: Thoroughly dissolve 1 heaping teaspoon of salt and 1 level teaspoon of baking soda in 1/2 cup of water. Stir well, and add to a 2-quart enema bag filled with warm water. Lie on your left side. The combination of salt and baking soda purifies and heals the lymph flow, reduces the tendency for acidity and prevents irritation and strengthens the colon by removing any fecal matter clinging to the colon walls.

If cramping occurs, stop the intake of water momentarily; continue at a slower intake speed when the cramping subsides. When all the water has been emptied into the colon, retain for 10-15 minutes before expelling.

Second bag: Repeat as above, but knee-chest position.

Third bag: Add 2 tablespoons of Glyco-Thymoline to the bag filled with warm water, and lie on your right side. Glyco-Thymoline reduces acidity, toxicity, fermentation, and cleanses and purifies. These are extremely important in restoring an unbalanced lymph system.

Contraindicated for people with heart, kidney, digestive and blood pressure problems. (Glyco-Thymoline is available through your pharmacy.)

Four Steps to Achievement:

Plan Purposefully

Prepare Prayerfully

Proceed Positively

Pursue Persistently

—William A. Ward

AWARENESS OF REDNESS

Any area of your lymphatic system that is compromised is not moving your interstitial fluid as readily as in the rest of your body. This stagnated fluid can be an invitation for bacteria in your system or entering via a cut in the skin to multiply, especially if the area becomes acidic. You may experience an inflammation or infection that can quickly become acute.

Cellulitis is an acute infection of the skin and subcutaneous tissue. The symptoms are as follows: your skin will feel hot to the touch and it will be red and painful, and swelling will occur along with fever, chills, uneasiness and headache. You will feel much like you are getting the flu.

Or you may experience erysipelas, an acute infection caused by A beta-hemolytic streptococci. This condition will be characterized by redness, swelling, vesicles, bullae, fever, pain and lymphadenopathy (swelling of lymph nodes or vessels). With the redness you will see red lesions on your skin.

Another condition that is associated directly with an inflammation of the lymphatic vessels is lymphangitis. When the inflammation involves only the lymphatic vessels it is called true lymphangitis. When an inflammation or infection is caused by bacteria or an allergic reaction, its involvement may include the lymphatic vessels along with other tissue. With other tissue involvement it will not be true lymphangitis.

Sometimes there may be a non-specific general inflammation to the area affected by a compromised lymphatic system. This is referred to as a "secondary acute inflammation," or S.A.I.

If you have had surgery that resulted in a compromised lymph system, causing stagnation of lymph, you are at life-time risk for one of the above-mentioned conditions. Seek medical help immediately if experiencing any of these conditions. Cellulitis in itself can be life-threatening and has caused a few of my clients to be admitted to the intensive care unit, for treatment with antibiotics.

If you are traveling to any remote location where medical care is not readily available you need take special precautions. It is advisable to travel with one or even two prescriptions of antibiotic, which you can self-administer in the event that you experience any of the above conditions and you are unable to immediately access a medical center.

What can you do while traveling to assist the body? Be mindful of the food combining rules. Be strict with the food combining early in the day if you're planning to go out for a large meal and dessert in the evening. Drink water – six to eight glasses each day to keep your body hydrated - it is the vehicle by which the lymph system moves material. This hydration will help prevent excess acidity from occurring in the tissue. Each and every day eat a large raw salad to alkalize the body and buffer acidity. If possible at the beginning of the day have the juice of half of a fresh lemon; this also will buffer acidity. Remember not to have any starch within an hour before or after having the lemon juice. You may put this in water to drink it, but be sure to rinse your mouth after as the citrus juice can be hard on tooth enamel. The goal is to buffer acids and keep the body slightly alkaline.

These food ideas will not guarantee that you will be able to avoid these conditions; however, they will make them less likely. Hopefully, they will allow you to enjoy your vacation rather than spend it at a medical center.

Lifestyle Recommendations

Don't ignore increased swelling, infection, redness, blistering, fever or inflammation of the affected area or body trunk. Call your doctor if the swelling persists or the symptoms do not improve.

Use the unaffected limb for blood pressure measurements, injections and blood drawing.

Shave hair from the affected limb with an electric razor only; change heads as necessary and keep the razor clean.

Light exercise is good for shorter, rather than longer periods, so as not to over-tire the limb. Walking is the best exercise - walk twenty minutes a day (exercising the muscles causes lymph flow).

Avoid any strenuous type of repetitive movements, such as raking, shoveling, or gardening.

Diuretic medications are contraindicated.

Avoid any product with Benzo-Pyrones, or with aluminum (i.e. antiperspirants) as these products may affect the lymph system.

Avoid wearing rings, watches or any tight jewelry. Avoid wearing socks, undergarments and bras that are elasticized, have narrow straps or underwire support. All clothing should be loose and comfortable, without tight constriction. Choose a light breast prosthesis.

Wear protective gloves for gardening, washing dishes and general cleaning. Avoid any trauma to the affected limb, including insect bites, cat scratches, burns, or bruising. Any hematoma (bruising) or trauma should be followed immediately by a MLD treatment.

Change position of the affected limb often; don't let it rest in any one position for too long. Carry your purse, shopping bags or other items with the unaffected arm. Consider a Healthy Back Bag, available through mail order companies.

Sleep so your body weight does not rest on the affected limb.

Avoid temperature extremes such as hot showers (use warm water for bathing) and direct sun (wear protective clothing or stay in a shaded area).

Avoid cutting the cuticles on the fingers and toes of affected limbs.

Wear your compression sleeve or bandages when traveling by air or during long ground travel. Get light exercise during your travel time, if possible. Keep your compression sleeve clean and have your garment corrected if any chaffing, redness or tightness occurs. Care for your compression sleeve as recommended by the manufacturer and replace as needed.

Skin care: Products such as Eucerine (choose the cream, which does not contain aluminum stearate) are available in most drug stores as a good moisturizing cream for the skin.

For a natural skin care lotion, mix 50% cold pressed olive oil and 50% cold pressed peanut oil with a few drops of lavender essential oil. This mixture will stimulate the circulatory and lymphatic system as well as provide maximum nourishment for the skin. You can purchase these items at health stores. Do not use peanut oil if you have a peanut allergy.

Breathing simulates the main lymph duct: Take four deep breaths, then take four regular breaths - repeat three times.

Have a massage for stress reduction each month - this will promote vascular function, lymphatic drainage, and nervous system coordination. **Caution:** Do not let the therapist do any deep tissue massage or vigorous work on the affected quadrant; only gentle strokes should be used. Use the natural skin care lotion mentioned above as the massage oil.

LYMPHATIC EXERCISES

Exercise I   Typical Morning Exercise

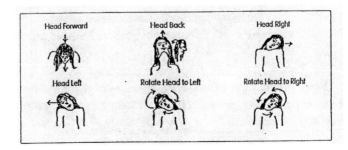

Exercise I: Bend the head forward three times, back three times, right three times and left three times. Then rotate the head left and right three times. Do these movements slowly, gently and with purpose. This will improve the circulation; stimulate the nerve plexus and lymph drainage of the head and neck area. Repeat this set four times.

Exercise II   Typical Morning Exercise

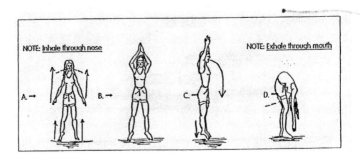

Exercise II Rise slowly up on the toes while inhaling through the nostrils; gradually raise the hands above and a bit forward of the head. Then slowly stand flat on the floor, bending at the waist and swinging the arms through the legs, forcefully expelling the air from the lungs through the mouth. Repeat slowly twelve times.

Exercise I   Typical Evening Exercises

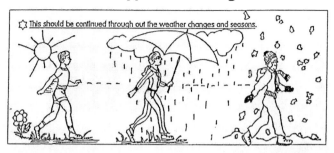

This should be continued through out the weather changes and seasons.

Exercise I: Walking does not place great strain on the body. Your calf muscles will act as great pumps returning blood and lymph to the heart. Swinging the arms help the circulation of the upper body. Walking will produce a gentle massage to the intestines which will help digestion. The recommended length of time is about a half an hour. It should be done after the evening meal to promote relaxation for a good nights sleep. If this is not possible, try to get your walk in during the lunch hour or by taking the stairs or by parking out in the parking lot.

Exercise II   Typical Evening Exercise

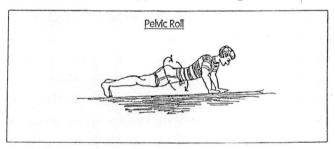

Pelvic Roll

Exercise II: Place the feet against the wall with the hands on the floor as like preparing for a pushup. Keeping your elbows relatively straight, rotate your trunk and hips, to the left and to the right, circle four times. Repeat these steps three times. Start this exercise gradually as it may be difficult at first. If this is too difficult you may stand in a doorway with the door open and grasp the moldings to steady your self. Keep your feet apart and rotate the hips left and right.

The best exercises are the ones you do each day. Moderate exercise is the goal.

Finding a Manual Lymph Drainage Therapist

Seeking out a qualified therapist to begin treatments can be difficult, depending on your local resources. There are a number of MLD training schools throughout the world, and you might want to begin looking for a therapist by contacting one of the following institutions:

The Dr. Vodder School International, (www.vodderschool.com) or (250-598-9862)

The North American Vodder Association of Lymphatic Therapy, (www.navalt.org) or (888-462-8258)

The Foeldi School (Germany), (www.foeldiklinik.de/index_ en.html) or Tel.: ++ 49 7652 - 124 - 0

The Casley-Smith School, (www.lymphoedema.org.au) or (www.casley-smith-lymphedema-courses.org) or send queries through the websites

The Klose Training and Consulting School, (www.klosetraining.com) or 303-245-0333

Wherever the therapist undertakes training, certain standards should be adhered to. The National Lymphedema Network Newsletter (www.lymphnet.org or 510-208-3200) suggests that the therapist have at least 80, but preferably 120, hours of training. Vodder method training (the original and unaltered method) requires 160 hours with 25 hours re-certification every two years.

When you do find a therapist, make sure that he or she is willing to spend at least 45 minutes or more in administering the Manual Lymph Drainage techniques. Don't be afraid to ask questions about your treatment, or to bring up any concerns you might have. Ultimately, you must feel comfortable with your therapist, and trust in their ability to help you along in the healing process.

As a client, you must also recognize the limitations of the therapist, and take responsibility for the role you play in the long-term management of your own health.

Self-Massage

Self-massage can play an integral role in keeping the tissue soft and pliable. There are videos available through the National Lymphedema Network (510-208-3200) and through the Dr. Vodder School (250-598-9862). With the help of the therapist from whom you are receiving treatment you can learn to self-massage correctly.

Bandaging Techniques

The benefits of Manual Lymph Drainage can be extended through the practice of compression bandaging following each treatment. Bandaging provides needed support to the affected limb by replacing the missing tissue pressure, and is preferred over compression garments in the early stages of treatment. Compression bandaging requires a specific technique to be effective and not cause harm, and should be attempted for the first time in the presence of your MLD therapist. He or she will be able to direct you as to the correct bandages to use, where and how to apply specific amounts of pressure, and the length of time the compression bandage should be worn.

Once you have a basic understanding of how compression bandaging should be practiced, you should use it after each MLD session. Some of the signs that you are applying the bandages incorrectly are a light bluish discoloration in the fingers or toes during or immediately after bandaging that does not vanish upon movement, and/or whitish discoloration in the fingers or toes.

If these symptoms appear, the area needs to be re-bandaged. If you are unable to apply the bandages without adverse results, review the technique with your therapist at your next appointment.

Various compression sleeves are available and can be instrumental in enhancing re-absorption of fluid. Consult your therapist for additional information.

Conclusion

Lymphedema is treatable with *Manual Lymph Drainage techniques, compression, friendly foods, exercise, and Light Beam Generator Therapy.* The short- and long- term results of the therapy will be dependent upon the skills and insight of the therapist and the willingness of the client to participate in his or her own therapy. Treatment success will also be affected by the genetic blue print of each client: the number of lymphatic vessels, their size, communication with the nervous system, back flow valve functioning, and the client's prior history of diet and exercise. One must also take into account the life-saving cancer treatments the client has undergone, including the extent of the surgery and of radiation treatment, and the impact that these treatments may have had on the lymphatic system.

It is clear that one must not look back. The focus should be on the future and on employing all of these tools to better your situation. Knowledge is power when it is put into action. Long-standing lymphedemas require patience and persistence. You can always improve your situation: thoughts will become words, and words will become deeds, which will lead to improvement. The human body is amazing. As we speak or sleep, it is constantly working to maintain its state of health, adjusting itself to any circumstance.

By removing the roadblocks that may prevent optimum health, through exercise, proper nourishment, and using all of the tools outlined in this book, you can take charge and help your body move toward a better state of health.

You now have the information you need to eat, exercise, and compress your limb to better health. With a personal commitment, nurture yourself. Take the first step now!

About Edgar Cayce

Edgar Cayce was born on a small farm near Hopkinsville, Kentucky in 1877. His childhood friends were seen only by him, and when questioned, he said these playmates were the spirits of deceased children. When having difficulties with his spelling lessons, he discovered that by sleeping with a book under his pillow, he could learn the lesson for the week and all the lessons in the book. After a particularly moving church service, he went to the woods with his Bible to pray to heal the sick. He was visited by a radiance that said he could if he remained faithful to his prayers.

Cayce began to experience psychic self-induced trance states as an adult. For forty years he gave these trance-like readings, and from these readings came medical diagnoses and treatment suggestions for thousands of people. Besides giving medical readings, he gave readings on dreams, meditation, reincarnation, prophecy, life, death and many other subjects.

By his death in 1945, he gave approximately 14,000 readings. These readings are archived at the Association for Research and Enlightenment (A.R.E.), located in Virginia Beach, Virginia, and are available to the public. There is also an A.R.E. Clinic in Phoenix, Arizona, where western and holistic medicine is used in the treatment of clients.

There is a River, by Thomas Sugrue, will further acquaint the reader with the Edgar Cayce story.

Further Readings

Baroody, Dr. Theodore A. *Alkalize or Die* Holographic Health Press 1999

Bolton, Brett. *Edgar Cayce Speaks of Foods, Beverages, and Physical Health* Avon Books 1969

Campbell PhD, T. Colin Campbell. The China Study

Casley-Smith, J.R. & Casley-Smith, Judith R. *High-Protein Oedemas and the Benzo-Pyrones*, Lippencott Company/Harper & Row 1986

Cayce, Edgar. Circulating File # 0271: Dropsey Edgar Cayce Foundation 1971

Cayce, Edgar. Readings pertaining to Calcios

Colbin, Annemarie. *Food And Healing* Ballantine 1986

Consumer Reports on Health July 1997 Too Little Sun?

Cook, John. *The Book of Positive Quotations* Fairview Press 1993

DuBelle, Lee. *Proper Food Combining Works* Lee DuBelle 1997

Duggan, Sandra, R.N. *Edgar Cayce's Guide to Colon Care* Inner Vision Publishing 1995

Feskanich D, Willett WC, Stampfer MJ, Colditz GA *American Journal of Public Health* 1997 Jun; 87(6):992-7 Milk, dietary calcium, and bone fractures in women: a 12-year prospective study

Feskanich D, Willett WC, Stampfer MJ, Colditz GA *American Journal Epidemiology* 1996 Mar 1;143 (5):472-9 Protein Consumption and Bone Fractures in Women

Foldi, Michael M.D. & Ethel, M.D. *Lymphodema Methods of Treatment and Control* Gustav Fischer Verlag 1991

Gabbay, Simone. *Nourishing the Body Temple* A.R.E. Press 1999

Gabbey, Simone. Venture Inward March/April 1999 Aromatherapy Offers Fragrant healing Energies.

Grabowski, Sandra Reynolds and Tortora, Gerard J. Principles of Anatomy and Physiology

Herbs for Health Cow's Milk: The Calcium Debate Sept/Oct 1998
Holistic Health Journal vol. 2 no. 3 Autumn 95 Osteoporosis: Sorting Fact From Fallacy

Kasseroller, Renato, M.D. *Compendium of Dr. Vodder's Manual Lymph Drainage* Haug International 1998

Keough, James, Alternative Medicine Magazine. Bones of Contention Ireland, Corydon, Harvard News Office. Hormones in milk can be dangerous

Kurz, Ingrid. *Textbook of Dr. Vodder's Manual Lymph Drainage: Volume 2 Therapy* 4th Edition Haug International 1997

Kurz, Ingrid. *Textbook of Dr. Vodder's Manual Lymph Drainage: Volume 3 Treatment Manual* 3rd Edition Haug International 1996

Liebman, Bonnie. *Nutrition Action* vol. 21 no. 5 Calcium: After the Craze

Marandino, Cristin. *Vegetarian Times* Got Milk-or More? November 1997

Mein, Eric M.D. *The New Millennium*, The Legacy of the Health Readings vol. 5 no. 3 June/July 2000 Association of Research and Enlightenment, Inc.

Melina, Vesanto & Messina, Virginia and Mark. *Herbs for Health* July 1997 Calcium Conclusions

Mills, Cynthia *Health* July/August 1999 Got Calcium?

Mosby's Medical, Nursing & Allied Health Dictionary, Fifth Edition Mosby Year Book, Inc. 1998

Nutrition Action vol. 24 no. 8 Vitamin D Deficiency-: The Silent Epidemic

Pennington, Jean A.T. *Food Values of Portions Commonly Used* Harper & Row 1989

Reilly, Dr. Harold J. & Brod, Ruth Hagy. *The Edgar Cayce Handbook For Health Through Drugless Therapy* Macmillan/Jove 1977

Triviera, Larry. *Alternative Medicine* May 2000 Shedding Light on Lymphatic Health

Vegetarian Times February 1994 For the Record: Calcium Competition

Weil, Andrew. *Self Healing* December 1998 Good Fats, Bad Fats

Weil, Andrew. *Self Healing* September 1999 Second Opinion: Is Milk a Must?

Wittlinger, Gunther & Wittlinger, Hildegard. *Textbook of Dr. Vodder's Manual Lymph Drainage* Volume I: Basic Course 5th Edition Haug International 1995

NOTES

NOTES

NOTES

CPSIA information can be obtained at www.ICGtesting.com
225902LV00003B/180/P

9 781608 445578